ROLLED LAMB BREAST RECIPE:

The Best Lamb Breast Recipe Grill For Beginners and Advanced Users

Lynnsey Crewell

TABLE OF CONTENTS

- INTRODUCTION 4
- Grilled Tandoori Chops 5
- Lamb Biryani 6
- Moroccan Lamb with Lemons and Olives 8
- French Style Roast Lamb 10
- Lamb Hot Pot 11
- Lamb Scotch Broth 13
- Lamb with mushroom sauce 14
- Barbecued Butterfly Lamb 16
- Stuffed Lamb Chops 18
- Strawberry Curried Lamb 19
- Sticky Dippy Lamb Chops 20
- Stewed Lamb Shanks & White Beans 21
- Stewed Chinese Lamb with Orange 23
- Spicy Orange Lamb 24
- Spicy Lamb Soup 26
- Spiced Grill-Pan Lamb Chops 27
- Special Roast Lamb 28
- Stuffed Leg of Lamb 29
- CONCLUSION 30

INTRODUCTION

Lamb breasts can be cooked in a variety of ways such as roasted, baked or grilled. It is a tough meat that needs slow and long cooking in order to tenderize it. Lamb meat contains lots of fat and thus it is suggested to avoid adding more fats to it while cooking or stuffing. Here is a lamb breast recipe to make a delicious dinner for you and your family.

What is the lamb breast recipes?

The ingredients that you need to make lamb breast include a whole breast of lamb, half can of diced tomatoes, half teaspoon of nutmeg, salt and pepper each, eight ounce pineapples, and two and half tablespoon of plain bread crumbs. Start with preheating the oven to 350 Fahrenheit. Add drained diced tomatoes, crushed pineapples, breadcrumbs, nutmeg, salt and pepper to a mixing bowl and mix together. You can add pineapple with juice to the bowl. The bone of the lamb breast is removed by the butcher.

Why Use the lamb breast recipes

Lay out the breast piece in such a way so as the side from where bone is removed is facing you. Spread the mixture over the breast piece and roll. Secure the meat in place with the help of a cooking string. Cut off the excess string and place the lamb breast in a roasting bag. Place the bag in a roasting pan. Make a few holes in the roasting bag to let the steam out. Place the pan in the oven. Twenty five minutes baking is enough for one pound of meat. As the stuffed breast take longer than usual so you must add twenty five more minutes to the usual time. Remove the lamb breast from the oven when done. Cut the string before serving your delicious lamb breast.

The recipe also includes vegetables in it that increases its nutritious value. Start with heating three tablespoon olive oil in a casserole dish over high heat. Cook the lamb breast to make it crispier from outside and seal the flavor inside. After cooking from both sides add chopped carrots, chopped celery, and a medium sized chopped onion to it. Sauté the veggies for three to four minutes and add three cloves garlic and rosemary to it. Pour vegetable or meat broth and half bottle of red wine in a casserole dish and cook. Allow the ingredients to simmer for 5 minutes on medium heat. Now place the casserole dish in the oven to cook for two and half hours at 150 degrees. Remove from the oven when done and serve hot.

GRILLED TANDOORI CHOPS

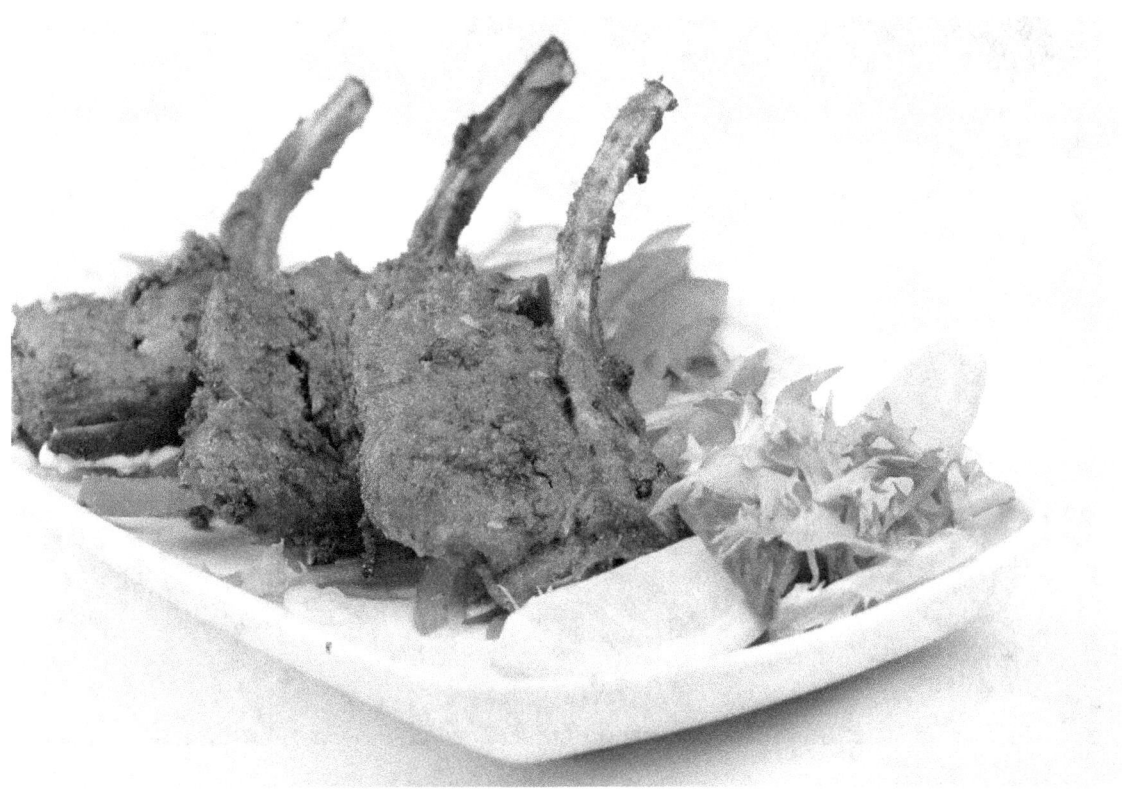

- 4 lamb or pork chops, each weighing 4 oz (110g)
- 2oz (50g) Greek Yoghurt
- 1 tablespoon bottled lemon juice
- 1 teaspoon bottled minced garlic
- ½ teaspoon chilli powder
- ½ teaspoon garam masala
- 1 tablespoon tandoori curry powder
- 1 tablespoon tomato puree
- ¼ teaspoon salt
- 4 tablespoons milk

1. Trim some, but not all, excess fat from the chops and make small gashes in the meat with a sharp knife.
2. Mix all the remaining ingredients into a paste in a non-metallic bowl.
3. Immerse the chops in the paste, ensuring they are well coated.
4. Preheat the frill to medium and line the frill tray with foil. Put the rack over it and the coated chops on the rack. Place the tray midway from the heat and grill the chops for about 5 minutes.
5. Turn the chops over and baste them with any spare paste. Grill for a minimum of another 3 minutes or until properly cooked.

LAMB BIRYANI

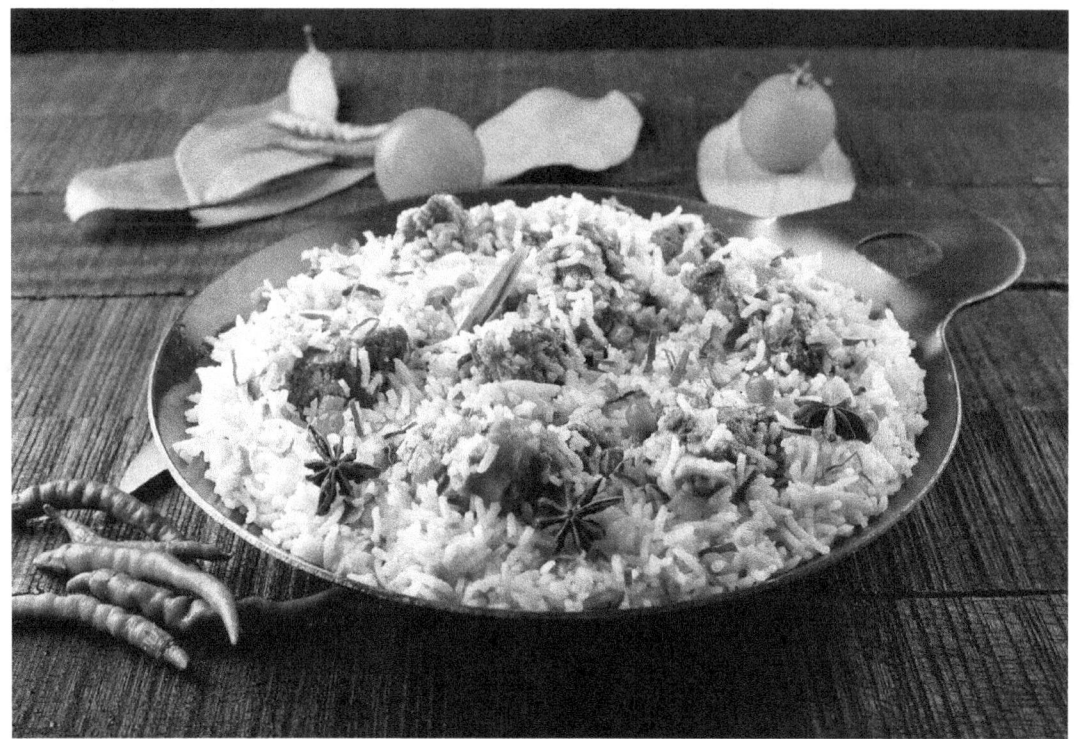

SERVES 6

- 450g (1 lb) white basmati rice
- slat
- 1 large onion
- 3 garlic cloves
- 6 cm (2 ½ inch) piece fresh root ginger
- 25 g (1 oz) flaked almonds
- 15ml (1 tbsp) ground coriander
- 10ml (2 tsp) ground cumin
- 5ml (1 tsp) ground fenugreek
- 700g (1 ½ lb) boned leg or shoulder of lamb
- 90 ml (6 tbsp) ghee or oil
- 1 cinnamon stick
- 6 green cardamoms
- 6 cloves
- 150ml (1/4 pint) thick yoghurt
- 5ml (1 tsp) saffron strands
- pinch of turmeric
- 40g (1 ½ oz) butter
- To Garnish:

- ❖ hard-boiled eggs
- ❖ sultanas
- ❖ toasted almonds
- ❖ garam masala
- ❖ coriander sprigs
- ❖ crisp-fired onions

1) Wash the rice in a sieve under cold running water until the water runs clear. Tip into a bowl, add 15ml (1 tbsp) salt and enough water to cover. Leave to soak for about 1 hour.

2) Peel the onion and cut into quarters. Peel the garlic. Peel and roughly chop the ginger. Put the onion, garlic, ginger, almonds and ground spices in a food processor or blender. Add 15 ml (1 tbsp) water and puree until smooth.

3) Trim the lamb of any excess fat and cut into 2.5 cm (1 inch) cubes. Heat the ghee or oil in a large flameproof casserole. Brown the lamb in batches over a high heat, adding more ghee or oil as necessary. Remove from the pan; set aside.

4) Add the onion and spice paste to the pan and cook over a fairly high heat for about 5 minutes until the paste is golden brown, stirring all the time. Add the whole spices and cook for a further 2 minutes. Return all the meat of the pan and stir to coat in the onion and spices.

5) Lower the heat and gradually add the yogurt a spoonful at a time, stirring constantly. Add 150 ml (1/4 pint) water, bring to a gentle simmer and coom for about 1 hour or until the meat is tender. Season with salt, cayenne and nutmeg. Cover with a tight-fitting lid and keep warm in a low oven set at 150c (300f) Mark 2 while cooking the rice.

6) Meanwhile, put the saffron in a small bowl with the turmeric and 60 ml (4 tbsp) warm water; leave to soak.

7) Drain the rice. Add to a large pan of boiling salted water, stir with a fork, then bring back to the boil and cook for 5 minutes. Drain thoroughly.

8) Pile the rice on top of the meat. Drizzle the saffron liquid across the rice and dot with the butter. Cover the casserole with a double thickness of foil, then the lid. Bake in the oven for 45 minutes.

9) To serve, transfer to a player, fluff the rice carefully with a fork and garnish with eggs, sultanas, almonds, garam masala, coriander and the crisp onions.

Note: For the crisp-fried onion garnish, fry 2 sliced large onions in oil until dark golden brown. Drain on kitchen paper.

MOROCCAN LAMB WITH LEMONS AND OLIVES

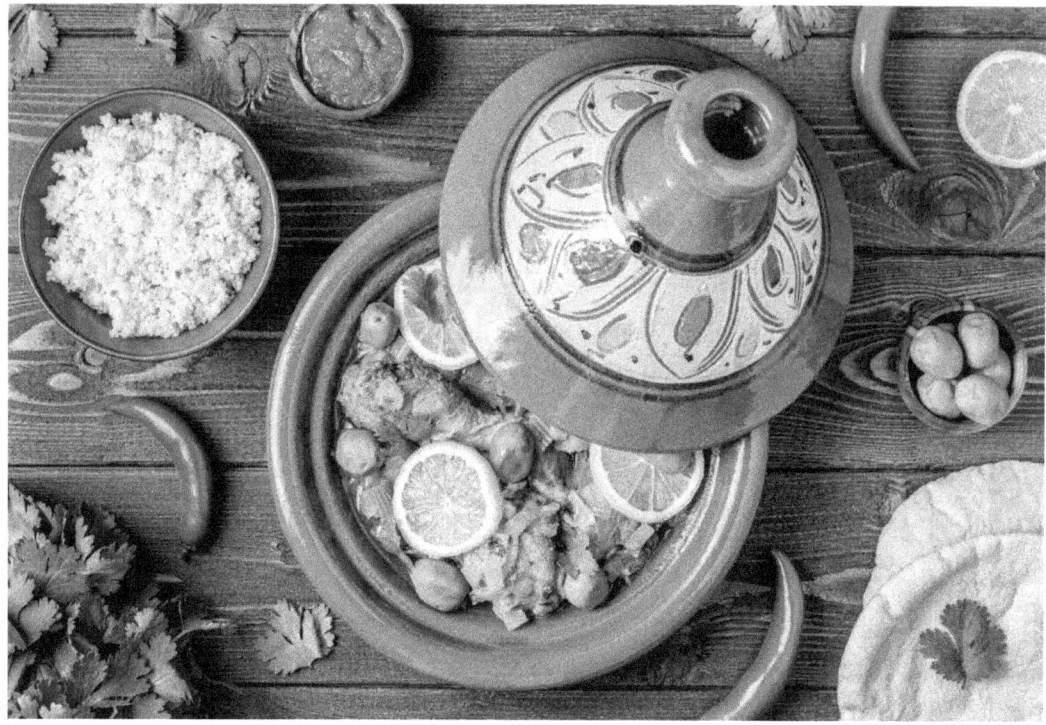

SERVES 6 CASSEROLE

- 1.4 kg (3 lb) boned leg or shoulder of lamb
- 2 large onions
- 3 large lemons
- 45 ml (3 tbsp) olive oil
- 45 ml (3 tbsp) Moroccan Spice Mixture
- 1 large bunch of flat-leaved parsley
- salt and pepper
- 225g (8 0z) green olives
- 1 red onion, to garnish

1) Trim the lamb of any excess fat and cut into 5 cm (2 inch) cubes. Peel and roughly chop the onions.

2) Pare a strip of rind from 1 lemon. Cu into shreds and set aside for the garnish.

3) Heat the oil in a flameproof casserole. Add the onions and cook over a fairly high heat for 2 minutes; remove from the pan. Quickly fry the meat in batches over a very high heat until nicely browned all over. Return all the meat and the onions to the casserole.

4) Add the spice mixture and cook, stirring all the time, for 2 minutes. Add 150 ml (1/4 pint) water and the juice of the pared lemon. Bring to the boil, then lower the heat. Cover with a lid and cook gently for about 1-1 ½ hours or until the lamb is really tender.

5) Meanwhile finely chop the parsley. Finely grate the rind from the two remaining lemons.

6) Add the olives to the casserole with the grated lemon rind and half of the parsley. Season with salt and pepper. Add a little more water if the liquid has completely reduced, but not too much 0 it should be fairly thick. Cook for a further 10 minutes.

7) Peel and chop the red onion. Taste and adjust the flavour of the casserole, adding more lemon juice if necessary. Serve sprinkled with the remaining parsley, red onion and shredded lemon rind.

FRENCH STYLE ROAST LAMB

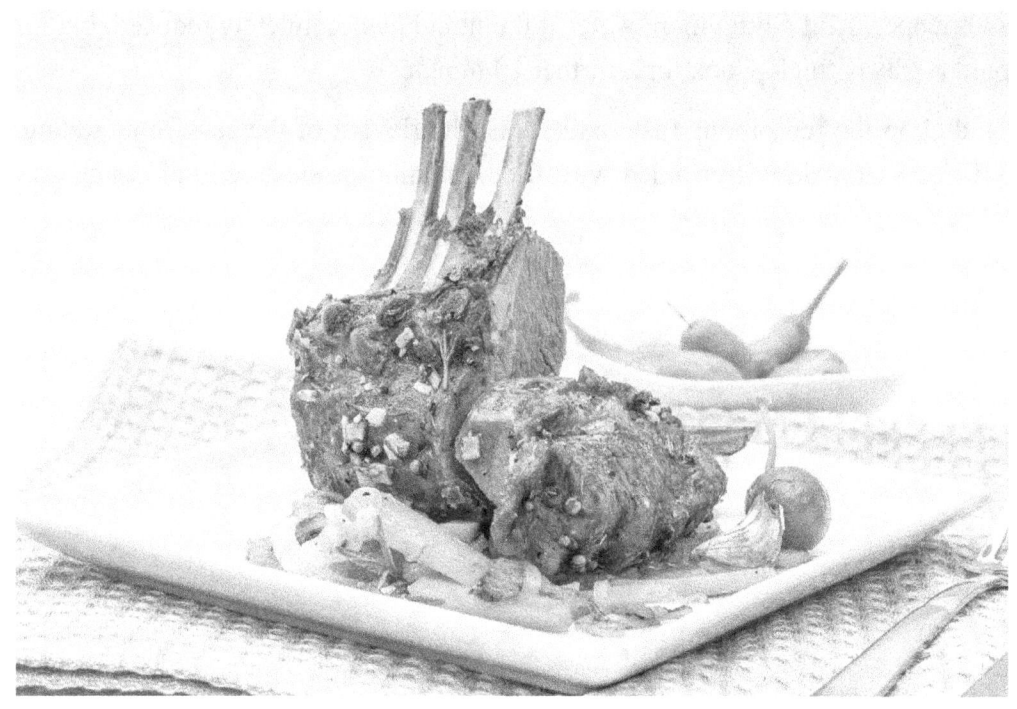

SERVES 4-6 COOKING TIME: 32 MINS APPROX

- 1.8-2kg/4-4 ½lb leg of lamb
- 4 tbls plum jam
- 3-4 garlic cloves, cut into spikes
- sprigs of fresh rosemary
- 6 plums, stoned and quartered
- 700g/ 1 ½lb cooked small potatoes, tossed in parsley and butter
- rosemary sprigs

1) Weigh the lamb and calculate the cooking time, 5-6 minutes per 450g /1 lb for rare, or 7-8 minutes per 450g / 1 lb for medium to well cooked lamb. Wipe the lamb, then make deep cuts over the surface of the skin, into the flesh. Brush with half the plum jam.

2) Stick garlic spikes and small pieces of rosemary into the cuts. Wrap a small piece of foil around the thin end of the lamb.

3) Place in a pierced roasting bag, and tie. Stand on a roasting rack and microwave on PL9 for half the calculated time.

4) Remove the roasting bag, brush with the remaining ham and cook for the remaining time. Leave to stand for 10 minutes, tented in foil. Place under grill to brown if wished.

5) Place plums in a bowl, cover with pierced film. Microwae on PL9 for 1 ½ minutes.

6) Arrange meat on a platter, and garnish with potatoes, plums and rosemary sprigs.

LAMB HOT POT

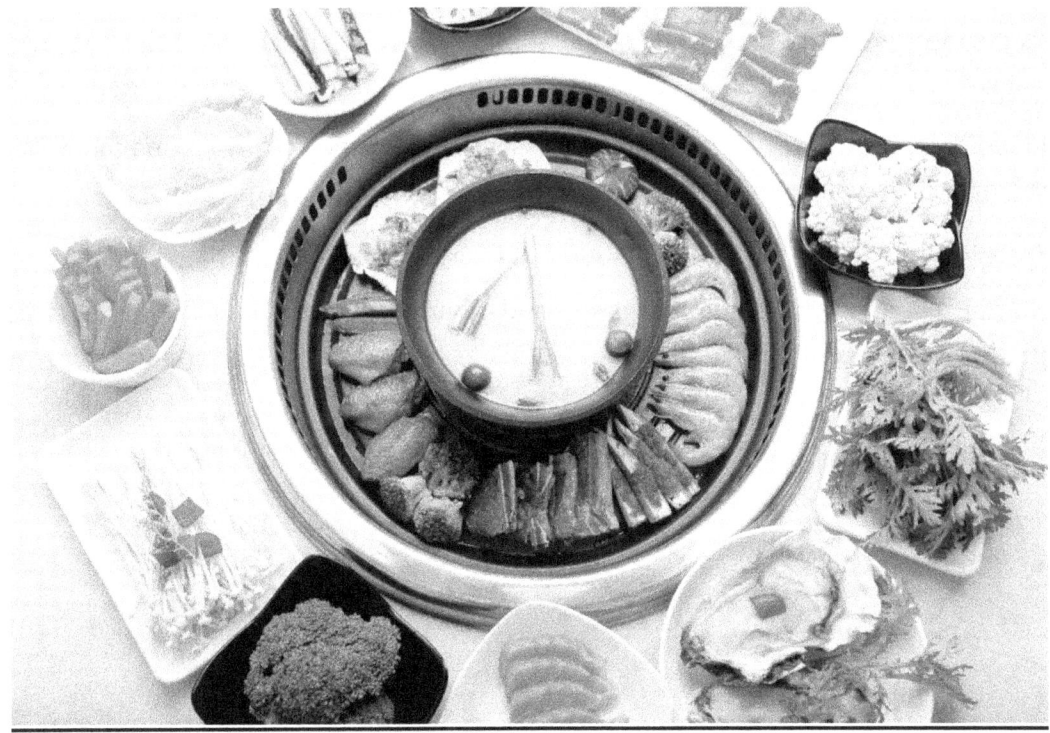

SERVES 4 COOKING TIME: 2 HOURS

- 450g / 1lb lean lamb cut into 2.5cm / 1in pieces
- 25g/1oz seasoned plain flour
- 25g/1oz butter or margarine
- 1 onion, chopped
- 1 garlic clove, curhsed
- 2 leeks, sliced
- 3 carrots, sliced
- 1 turnip, cubed
- 1 aubergine, chopped
- 400g / 14 oz can tomatoes
- 300ml/½pt hot beef or lamb stock
- bay leaf
- salt and pepper

Dumplings:

- 25g/1oz margaine50g/2oz self-raising flour
- 1 tbls chopped fresh herbs
- salt and pepper
- cold water to mix

To garnish:

- ❖ Fresh bay leaf

1) Toss the meat in the flour, then add to a 2.3L/4pt casserole with the fat. Microwave on PL9 for 3 minutes.

2) Add the onion, garlic, leeks, carrots, turnip, aubergine, canned tomatoes and juice, stock and bay leaf. Stir well, cover and microwave on PL9 for 10 minutes.

3) Reduce to PL4 for 10 minutes then PL2 for 1¼ hours. Stir.

4) Make the dumplings: rub the margarine and flour together, stir in the herbs, seasoning and sufficient cold water to mix. Add teaspoonfuls to the hot pot, re-cover and microwave on PL4 for 15 minutes.

5) Remove bay leaf, season and serve garnished with a bay leaf.

LAMB SCOTCH BROTH

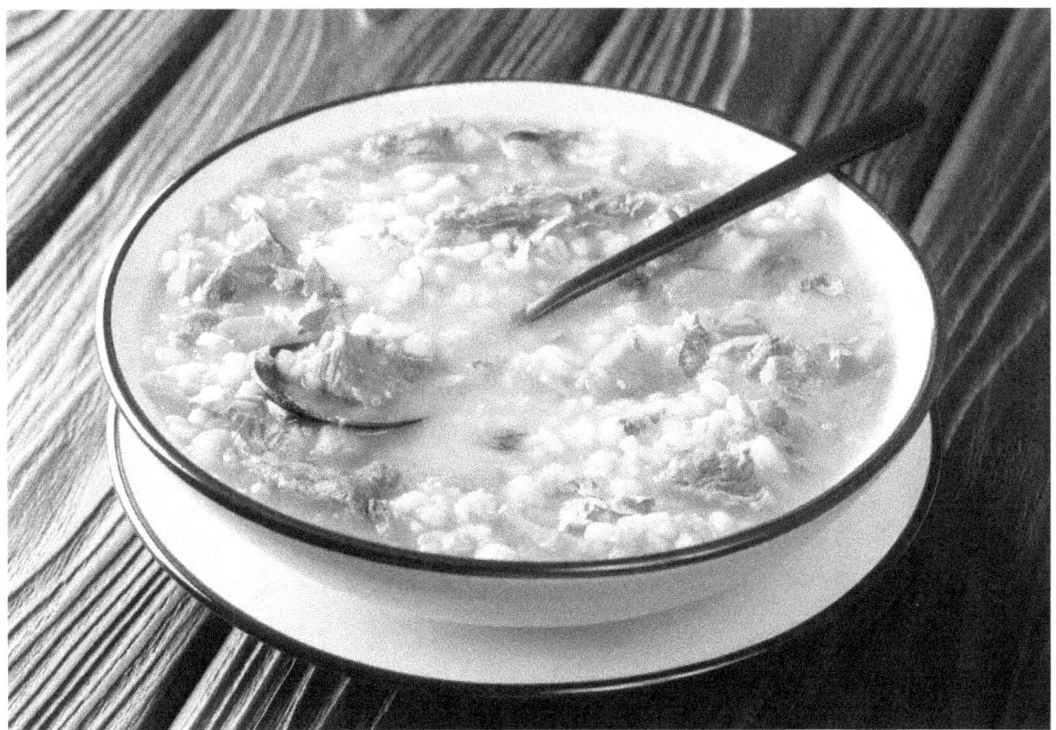

SERVES 4 COOKING TIME: 2 HOURS

- 700g (1 ½ lb) neck of mutton or shin of beef
- salt and freshly ground pepper
- 1 carrot, peeled and chopped
- 1 turnip, peeled and chopped
- 1 onion, skinned and diced
- 2 leeks, trimmed, thinly sliced and washed
- 45ml (3 tbsp) pearl barely
- 15ml (1 tbsp) chopped fresh parsley, to garnish

1) Remove any fat from the meat and cut the meat into bite-sized pieces. Put the meat in a saucepan, cover with 2.3 litres (4 pints) water, then add salt and pepper to taste. Bring slowly to the boil, cover and simmer for 1½ hours.

2) Add the vegetables and the barley. Cover and simmer for about another hour until vegetables and barley are soft.

3) Remove any fat that has formed on the surface with a spoon or absorbent kitchen paper.

4) Taste and adjust the seasoning of the soup, then serve hot, garnished with parsley. Traditionally, the meat is served with a little of the broth as a main course.

LAMB WITH MUSHROOM SAUCE

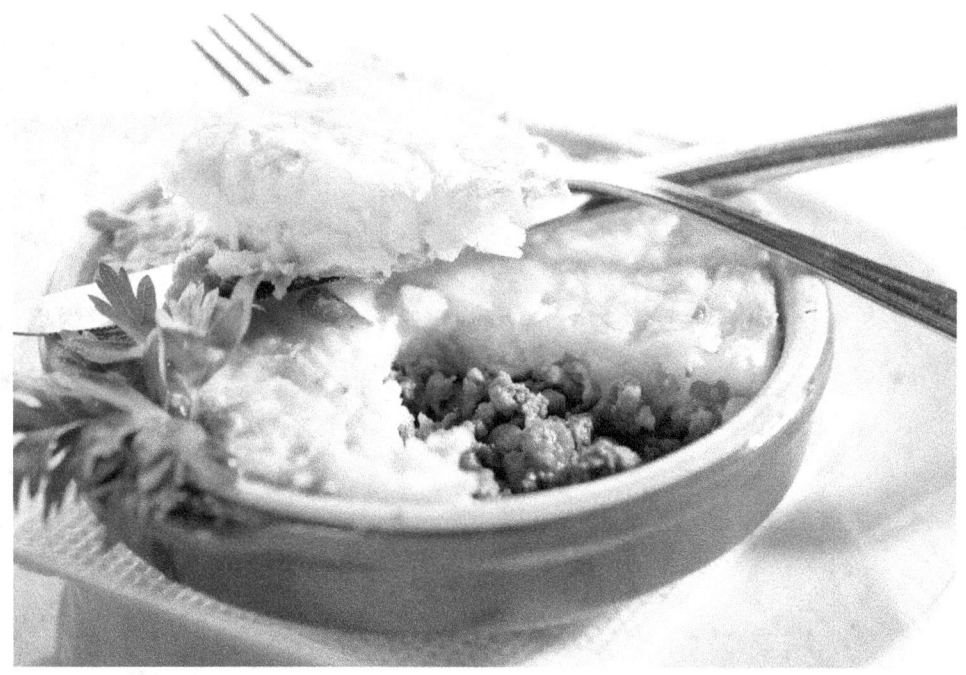

SERVES 6 PREPERATION TIME: 5MINS
COOKING TIME: 10 MINS

- 350g/12pz lean boneless lamb, such as fillet or loin
- 2 tbsp vegetable oil
- 3 garlic cloves, crushed
- 1 leek, sliced
- 175g/6oz large mushrooms, sliced
- ½ tsp sesame oil
- fresh red chillies, to garnish

Sauce

- 1 tsp cornflout (cornstarch)
- 4 tbsp light soy sauce
- 3 tbsp Chinese rice wine or fry sherry
- 3 tbsp water
- ½ tsp chilli sauce

1) Using a sharp knife or meat cleaver, cut the lamb into thin strips.

2) Heat the vegetable oil in a preheated wok or large frying pan (skillet).

3) Add the lamb strips, garlic and leek and stir-fry for about 2-3 minutes.

4) To make the sauce, mix together the cornflour (cornstarch), soy sauce, Chinese rice wine or dry sherry, water and chilli sauce and set aside.

5) Add the sliced mushrooms to the wok and stir-fry for 1 minute.

6) Stir in the prepared sauce and cook for 2-3 minutes, or until the lamb is cooked through and tender.

7) Sprinkle the sesame oil over the top and transfer the lamb and mushrooms to a warm serving dish. Garnish with red chillies and serve immediately.

BARBECUED BUTTERFLY LAMB

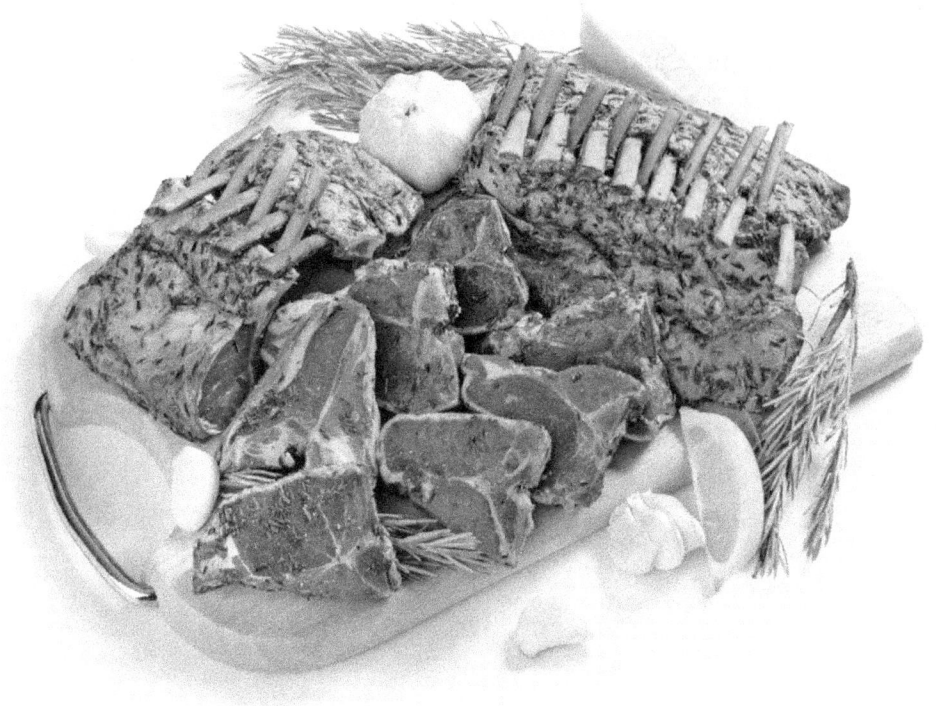

SERVES 4

PREPERATION TIME: 6¼ HOURS

COOKING TIME: 1 HOUR

- ❖ Boned leg of lamb, about 1.8kg/4lb
- ❖ 8 tbsp balsamic vinegar
- ❖ grated ring and juice of 1 lemon
- ❖ 150ml/¼pt/ 2/3 cup sunflower oil
- ❖ 4 tbsp chopped, fresh mint
- ❖ 2 cloves garlic, crushed
- ❖ 2 tbsp light muscovado sugar
- ❖ salt and pepper

To serve:
- ❖ Grilled (broiled) vegetables
- ❖ Green salad leaves

1) Open out the boned leg of lamb so that its shape resembles a butterfly. Thread 2-3 skewers through the meat in oder to make it easier to turn on the barbecue (grill).

2) Combine the balsamic vinegar, lemon rind and juice, oil, mint, garlic, sugar and salt and pepper to taste in a non-metallic dish that is large enough to hold the lamb.

3) Place the lamb in the dish and turn it over a few times so that the meat is coated on both sides with the marinade. Leave to marinate for at least 6 hours or preferably overnight, turning occasionally.

4) Remove the lamb from the marinade and reserve the liquid for basting.

5) Place the rack about 15cm/6in above the coals and barbecue (grill) the lamb for about 30 minutes on each side, turning once and basting frequently with the marinade.

6) Transfer the lamb to a chopping board and remove the skewers.

STUFFED LAMB CHOPS

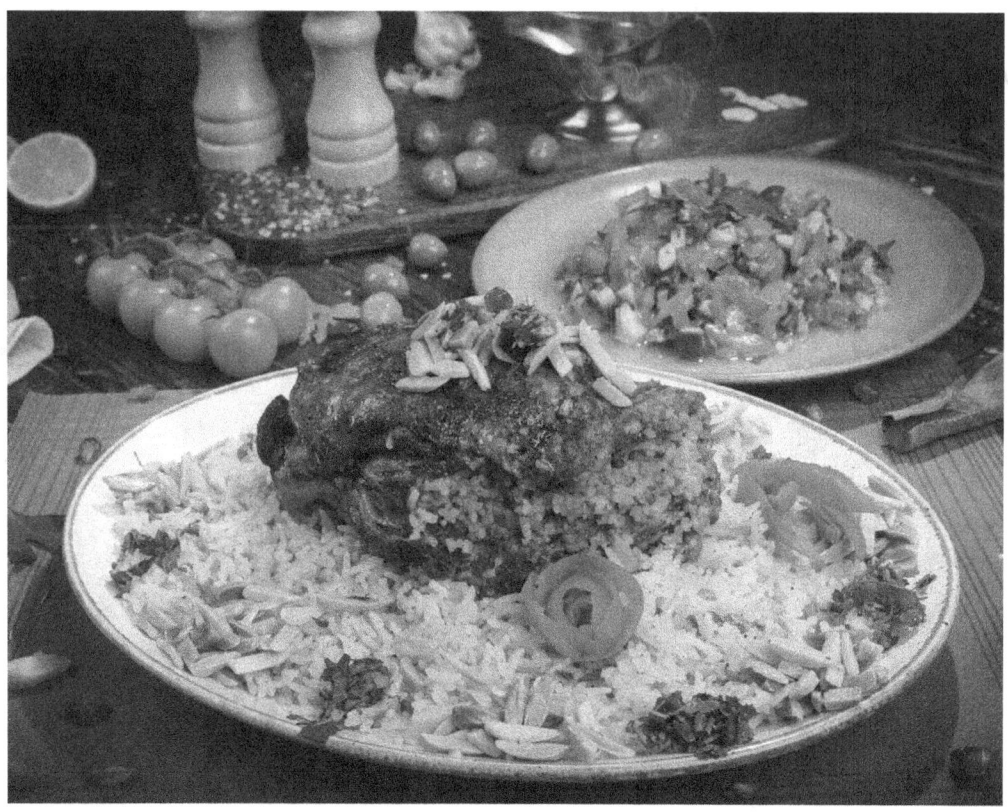

Ingredients:

- 4 American Lamb chops, 2 "thick With a pocket cut in the middle
- 8 pieces sourdough bread
- 1/4 lb sausage meat
- 2 pieces celery diced small
- 1 egg
- 1/8 tsp baking powder
- 1/4 cup chicken broth
- 2 Tbsp butter
- 3 Tbsp brown minute rice (cooked)
- 1 scallion, chopped
- 1/8 tsp ground cloves

Methods:

1) Mix this dressing together and then stuff it into the slot in the side of the lamb chop. Next on the top place a strip of bacon on the top in an "X" pattern. Top with a little Salt and fresh ground

2) pepper, garnish with fresh mint leaves Broil 8 minutes for rare, 14 minutes for medium rare, 18 minutes for medium.

STRAWBERRY CURRIED LAMB

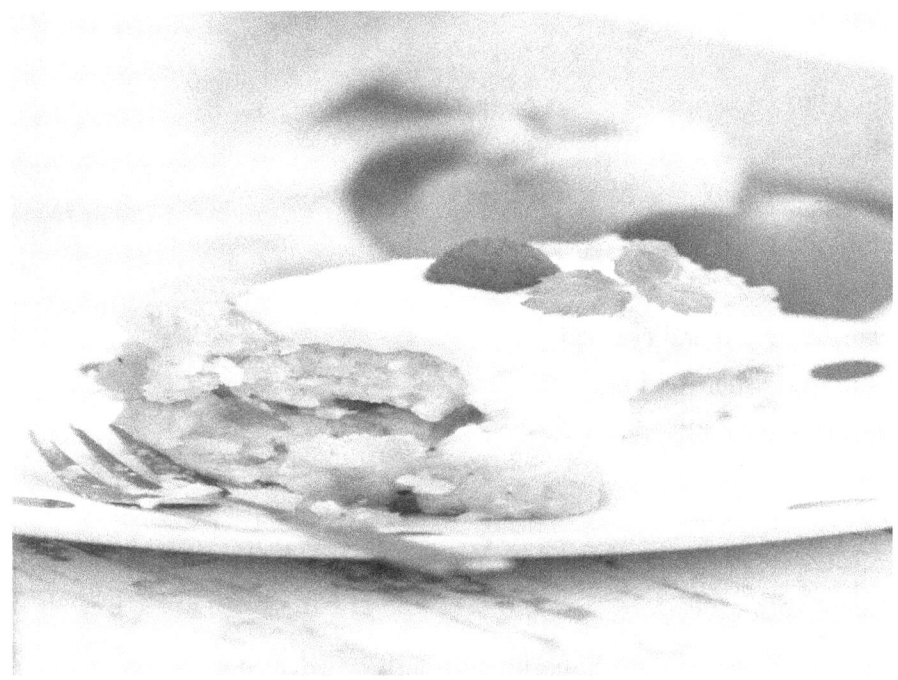

Ingredients:

- 3 cups (750 ml) fresh strawberries
- 1 tbsp (15 ml) all-purpose flour
- 1 tbsp (15 ml) curry powder
- ½ tsp (2 ml) dried thyme
- 1/4 tsp (1 ml) salt
- 1 lb (500 g) lean Ontario lamb, cubed
- 2 tbsp (25 ml) vegetable oil
- 1 medium onion
- 1 clove garlic, minced
- 3/4 cup (175 ml) diagonally sliced celery
- ½ cup (125 ml) chicken stock
- ½ cup (125 ml) plain yogurt or sour cream

Methods:

1) Puree 1 cup (250 ml) of the strawberries leave remaining berries whole or halve larger ones. Set aside. Combine flour, curry, thyme and salt toss lamb cubes in flour mixture to coat reserving any remaining flour mixture. In large skillet, heat oil over medium-high heat saute lamb, onion, garlic and celery for about 3 minutes or until lamb is browned. Sprinkle with remaining flour mixture stir in chicken stock and pureed strawberries. Reduce heat cover and simmer stirring occasionally, over low heat until lamb is tender about 20 minutes. Stir in yogurt. Add reserved whole strawberries and heat through.

STICKY DIPPY LAMB CHOPS

Ingredients:

- 8 lamb loin chops
- 1 Tbsp oil
- 5 Tbsp tomato ketchup
- 3 Tbsp runny honey
- 2 Tbsp dark soy sauce
- 2 cloves garlic, peeled and crushed
- 1 tsp mild chili powder (optional)
- 1 pot sour cream and chive dip

Methods:

1) Heat the oil in a large frying pan and fry the chops over a medium heat for 4-5 minutes on each side until nicely browned.

2) Mix the ketchup, honey, soy sauce, garlic and chili powder (if using) in a bowl. Stir the ketchup mixture into the pan and heat until bubbling. Cook for a further 2-3 minutes turning the chops once or twice, until the sauce is thick sticky and coats the meat.

STEWED LAMB SHANKS & WHITE BEANS

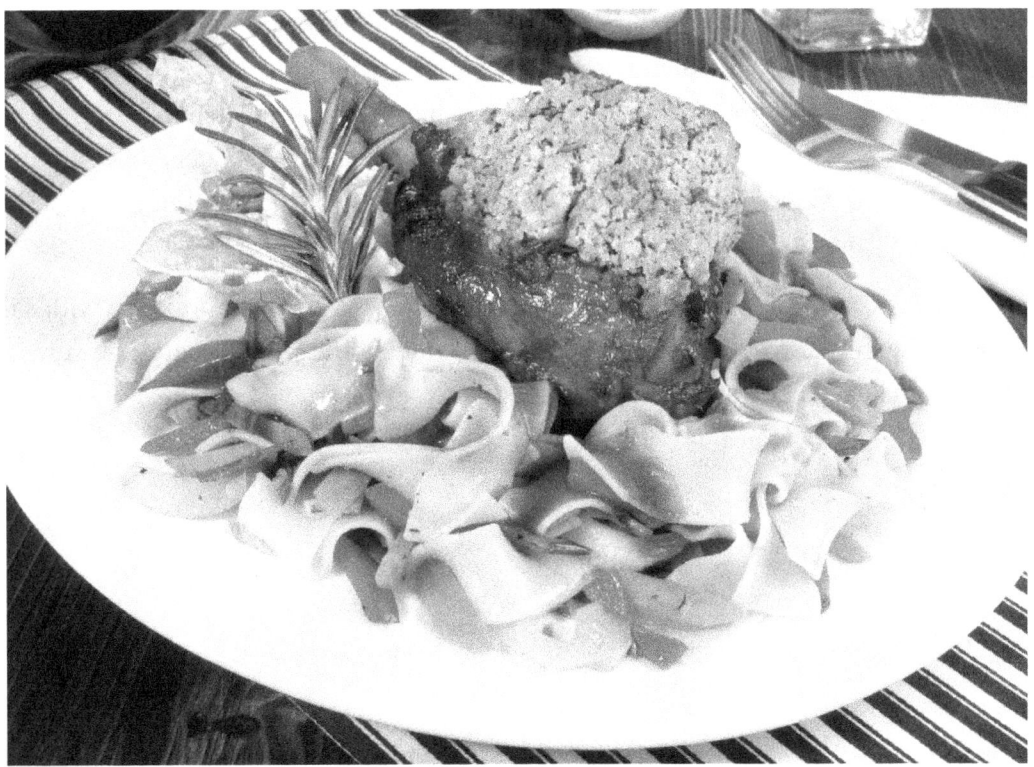

Ingredients:

- 8 Each Lamb Shanks, about 1 Lb Each — bones cracked
- 4 Teaspoons Kosher Salt
- Ground Black Pepper — to taste
- 5 Cloves Garlic — minced
- 1 Large Onion — diced
- 4 Medium Carrots — diced
- 3 Stalks Celery — diced
- 1 Cup Dry Red Wine
- 28 Ounces Can Whole Tomatoes In Puree
- 1 Pound Dried Great Northern Beans
- 8 Cups Chicken Broth
- 3 Sprigs Fresh Rosemary
- 2 Each Bay Leaves

Methods:

1) Soak the beans overnight in water to cover and drain or use the "quick soak" method. Season lamb shanks with 1 tsp of the salt and pepper to taste. In a large deep skillet, heat the olive oil

over medium-high heat. Add the lamb shanks on all sides about 10 minutes (.Do not crowd and work in batches if needed, removing fat as necessary).

2) Remove browned shanks to a platter. Add the garlic, carrots, onions and celery to the skillet and cook until softened, about 10 minutes. Pour in the wine and cook for 2 minutes. Transfer mixture to a large stockpot. Add the tomatoes using the back of a spoon to break up. Add the beans,shanks,stock, rosemary and bay leaves. Bring to a boil reduce to a simmer and skim surface as needed. Cover and cook until lamb and beans are tender about 2 hours.Skim as much fat as possible from the surface.

3) Remove shanks, using tongs, to 8 individual plates.Season the bean mixture with salt & pepper if needed.Discard the rosemary and bay leaves.Using a slotted spoon,arrange some of the bean mixture around each lamb shank.Serve immediately.

STEWED CHINESE LAMB WITH ORANGE

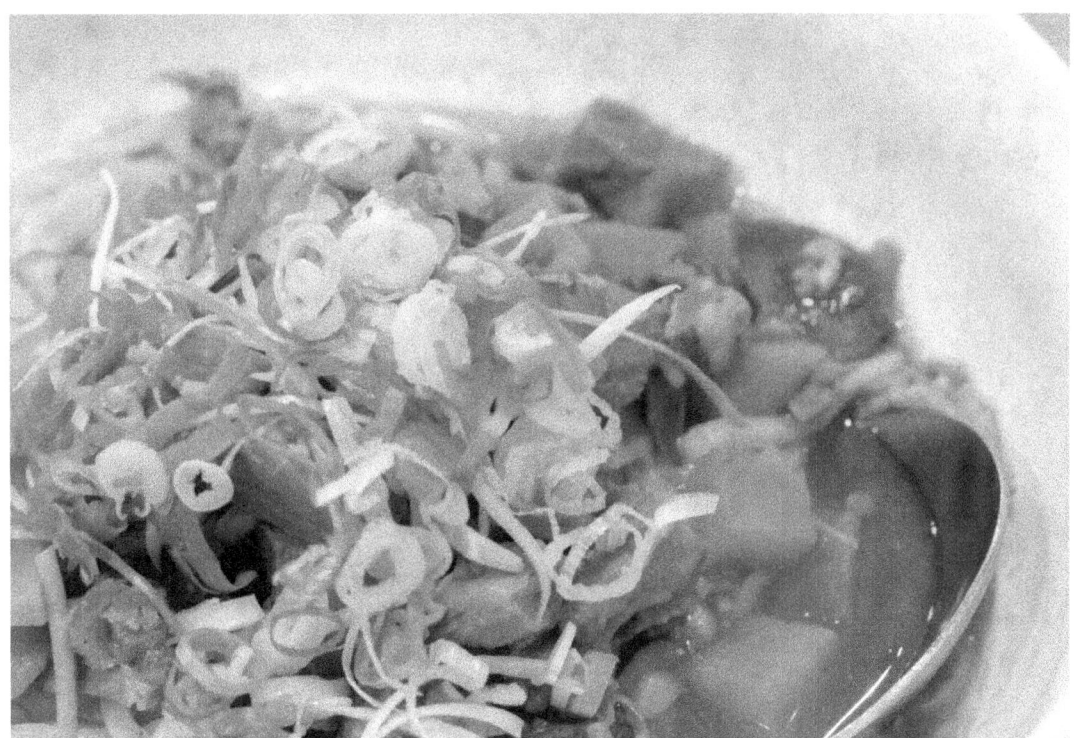

Ingredients:

- 2 lb lean lamb or mutton
- 1 tblsp soy sauce
- 1 tblsp sherry
- 1 tsp ground ginger
- 2 tblsp finely grated orange rind
- 1 tsp salt
- 1 litre stock or water
- 1 tblsp cornstarch

Methods:

1) Wipe the meat then cut into 1/2 inch cubes. Mix the soy sauce, sherry, ginger, orange rind and salt together add the lamb and mix well. Put the lamb into a pan with the flavorings and water. Bring to the boil remove the scum cover and simmer for 2 hours.

2) Mix the cornstarch to a smooth paste with a little cold water and add to the pan. Bring back to the boil stirring until slightly thickened.

SPICY ORANGE LAMB

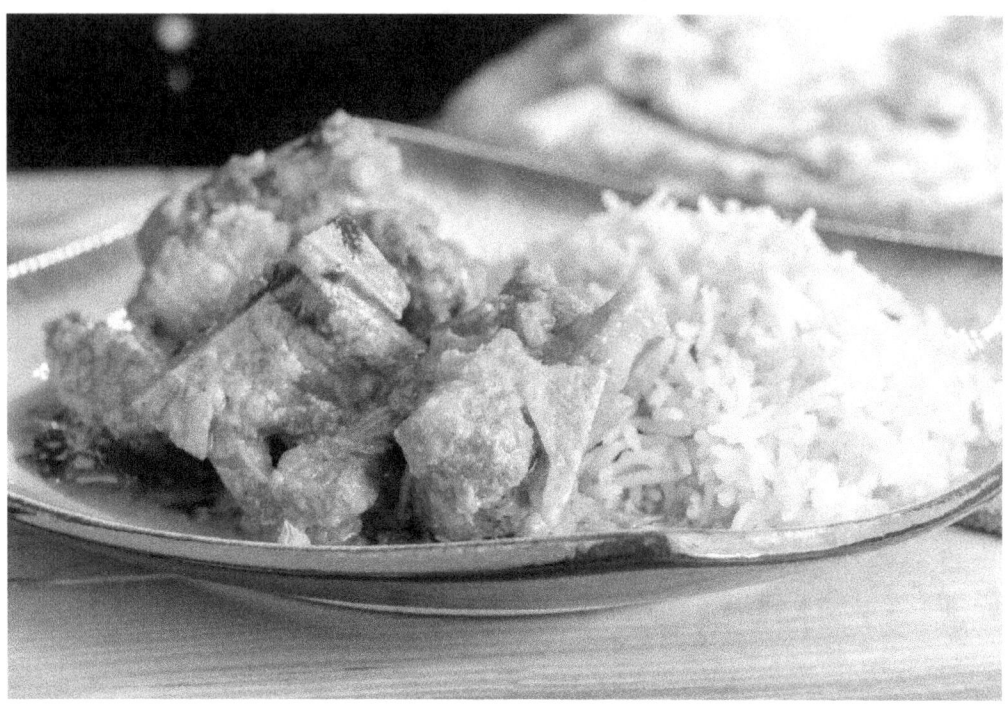

Ingredients:

- 450 g Lamb chops lean boneless
- 3 tbs Groundnut oil
- 1 1/2 ts Ginger root finely chopped
- 2 tbs Garlic thinly sliced
- 1 tbs Orange jest grated
- 1 ts Szechuan pepper
- 2 tbs Orange juice
- 1 tbs Dark soy sauce
- 2 ts Chili bean sauce
- 1/2 ts Salt
- 1/2 ts Freshly ground black pepper
- 1 ts Sugar
- 2 ts Sesame oil
- Marinade
- 1 tbs Light soy sauce
- 2 ts Rice wine or dry sherry
- 1 ts Sesame oil
- 2 ts Cornflour

Methods:

1) Roasted and finely ground (optional). "Here I have combined the lamb with orange for a lovely contrast to the rich meat. It is an easy dish to make and the spicy flavors add to its appeal.

2) Cut the lamb into thin slices 5cm long, cutting against the grain. Put the lamb into a bowl together with the marinade ingredients. Mix well and leave for about 20 minutes.. Add it to the pan and stir fry it for 2 minutes until it browns.

3) Pour off all but about 2 teaspoons of the oil. Stir-fry for 20 seconds. Then return the lamb to the pan, add the rest of the ingredients and stir fry for 4 minutes, mixing well. Serve the dish at once.

SPICY LAMB SOUP

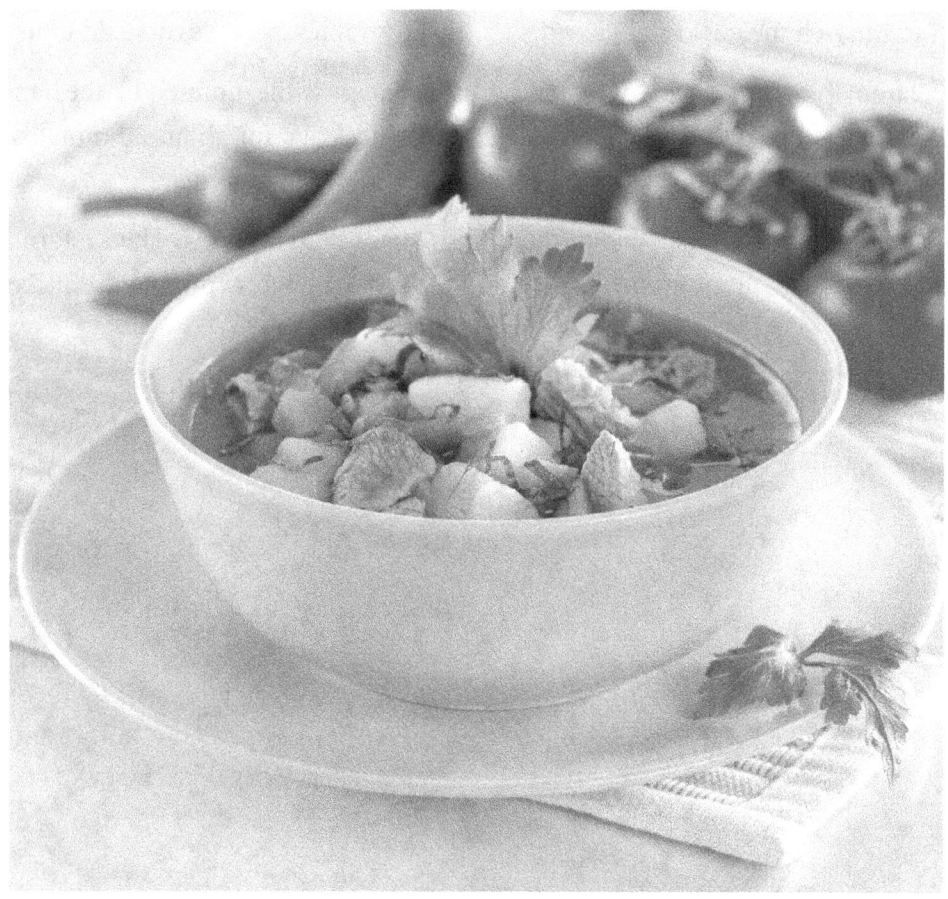

Ingredients:

- lamb fat (trimmings from a rack of lamb)
- ½ onion, chopped
- 1 tsp ground cinnamon
- 1 tsp curry powder
- 1 garlic clove, finely chopped
- one-third packet okra
- 2 tomatoes, chopped
- 1 beef stock cube
- 250ml/8fl oz water, boiling
- handful fresh soft herbs e.g. chives, parsley and basil

Methods:

1) Dice the lamb fat and melt in a pan. Add the onion and fry for 2 to 3 minutes until soft. Add the cinnamon, curry powder and garlic and fry for 2 minutes. Remove the tops from okra and chop into 1cm/½ inch pieces. Add okra and tomato to the pan. Dissolve stock cube in water and add to the soup. Simmer for 8 minutes. Roughly chop the herbs, stir them into soup and serve.

SPICED GRILL-PAN LAMB CHOPS

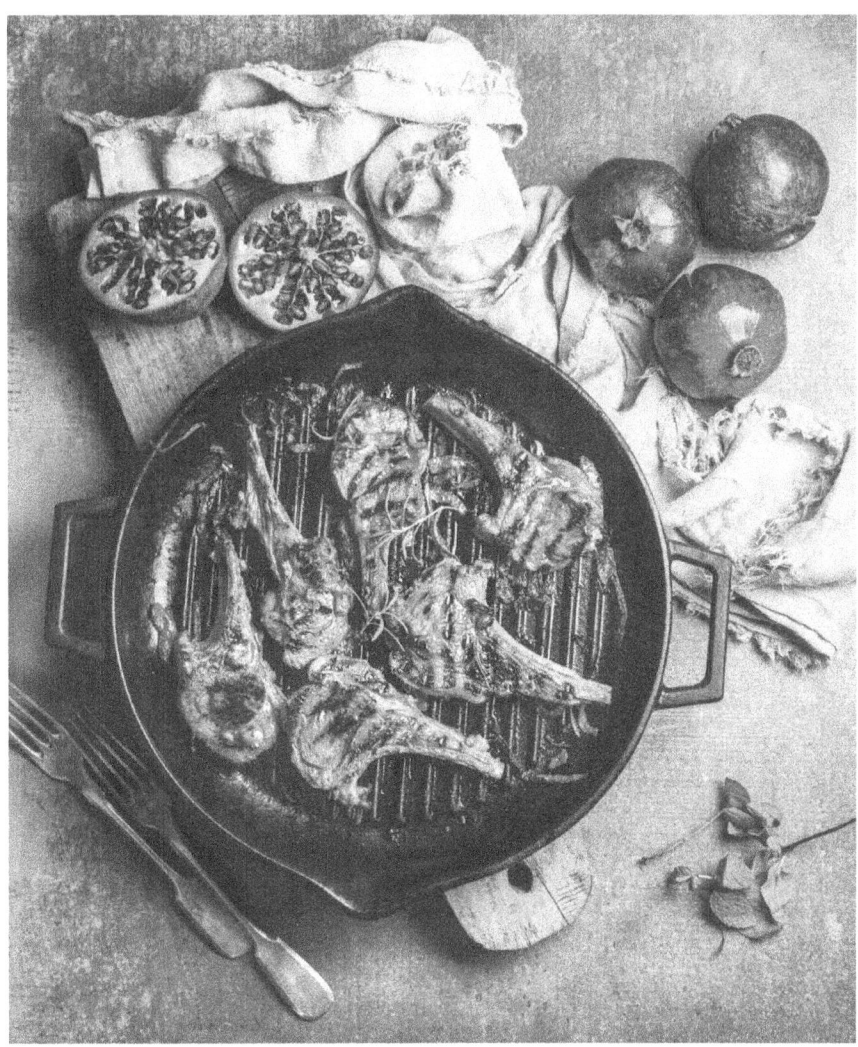

Ingredients:

- ❖ 1 tbs Cumin
- ❖ 1 ts Coriander
- ❖ 1/2 ts Salt
- ❖ 1/4 ts Freshly ground pepper
- ❖ 8 Bone-in loin lamb chops -trimmed

Methods:

1) Heat a large cast-iron grill pan over medium-high heat 10 minutes. Meanwhile heat a small skillet over medium heat. Toast cumin and coriander, 1 to 2 minutes. Combine with salt and pepper rub spice mixture over both sides of chops. Lightly coat the grill pan with vegetable cooking spray. Add 4 chops and cook 6 minutes per side for medium-rare. Transfer to plate; cover and keep warm. Repeat the process with remaining chops.

SPECIAL ROAST LAMB

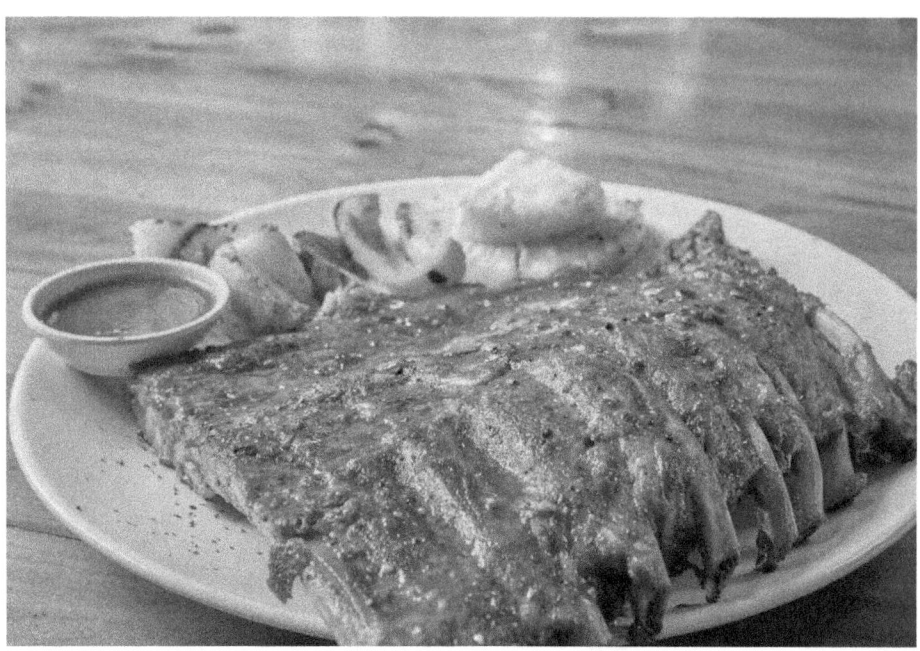

Ingredients:

- 5- to 6-lb (2.2- to 2.4-kg) lamb leg
- 1 tsp (5 mL) salt
- 1 tsp (5 mL) grated onion
- 1/4 tsp (1 mL) pepper
- 1/4 bay leaf, crushed
- 1/4 tsp (1 mL) ginger
- 1/4 tsp (1 mL) thyme
- 1/4 tsp (1 mL) sage
- 1 tbsp (15mL) salad oil (olive oil)

Methods:

1) Preheat oven to 325 F (160 C). Wipe lamb; cut small gashes 1/4-inch (0.5-cm) long on the top surface. Combine all ingredients except oil; rub mixture well into meat so that all the gashes are completely filled. Brush with oil. Place on rack in roasting pan. Bake in moderate oven until tender. Do not baste, cover or add water to the pan.

STUFFED LEG OF LAMB

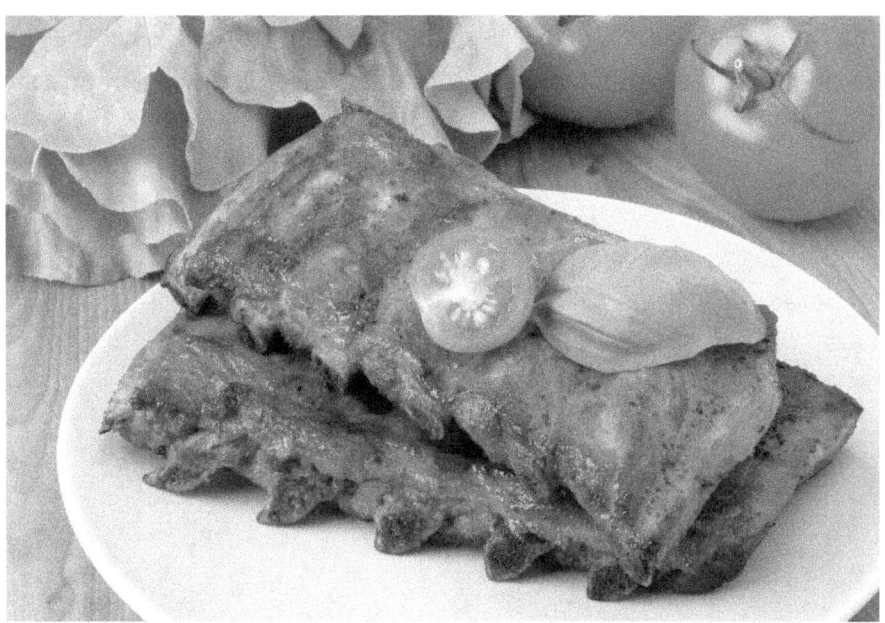

Ingredients:

- 5 pound boneless leg of lamb
- Smashed peeled garlic
- 2 teaspoons chopped fresh rosemary
- Stuffing (see recipe above)
- 1/4 cup red wine
- 3/4 cup brown stock or beef broth
- 1 pound peeled, seeded and chopped tomatoes
- 1 tablespoon slivered pitted olives
- Chopped parsley

Methods:

1) Preheat the oven to 400 degrees. Rub lamb inside and out with garlic clove. Stuff leg of lamb and tie securely sprinkle meat with rosemary.

2) Remove from oven as you finish sauce.

3) Discard fat in roasting pan. Add wine and broth and reduce. Add tomatoes and olives and season to taste with salt and pepper. Remove from heat add parsley

CONCLUSION

When buying young lamb, look for meat that is pink, firm and textured. When buying older lamb, the cuts should be lean and light red. Although a cross section of the bone will appear dried than that of young lamb, it should still be hard and red.

www.ingramcontent.com/pod-product-compliance
Lightning Source LLC
Chambersburg PA
CBHW080448220526
45465CB00007B/2804